5 Minute Parents: Small Habits, Big Impact

Naresh Kakerla

While every effort has been made to ensure the accuracy of the information contained in this book, the author and publisher assume no responsibility for errors, omissions, or any consequences arising from the use of the information provided.

5 Minute Parents: Small Habits, Big Impact Copyright © 2024 by Naresh Kakerla

ISBN: 9798345318560

Written by Naresh Kakerla

Introduction

In the present time, parents are so engrossed in their lives that they try desperately to be part of their kids' lives and realization is not very pronounced. 5 Minute Parents: Small Habits, Big Impact Enables this transformational change by tackling the belief that there needs hours of undivided attention in order to be a successful parent.

We are all quite aware about parent-child relations and significance of quality time. However, the demands of work, family and self-care almost always make parents feel bad or stressed. Not only does this book tell you the different things we think are quality time, but it provides evidence that it is not quantity, rather quality — how we spend our time with our children, what we do then and always looking for teachable moments — base. Creating connections, love and support and understanding from parents will help them to build stronger relationships with their children in a time where everything is chaotic so their children are made aware they feel valued and cared for.

Core Philosophy

It was a simple, yet resonant idea at the heart of "5 Minute Parents" — that small consistent habits can reap great dividends for kids' development and family life fundamentally. By spreading out short dose interactions in the course of a day, you set-up an environment for emotional intelligence, creativity and lifelong learning. Such an approach recognizes the ways in which family life has changed and supports us with tools to make every minute with our children as productive as possible.

Unique Approach

Instead of child-rearing guides that overwhelm with smothering long-term techniques or weekly practices that take time to complete, "5 Minute Parents" delivers quick little strategies, designed for even the busiest lifestyles. This collection of low-lift, do-it-now ideas are structured to build healthy relationships and maintain routines that benefit families through long-term habits.

5 MINUTE PARENTS: SMALL HABITS, BIG IMPACT

Key Concepts

Consistency: Children crave the sense of safety and trust that small, regular interactions can create. All these fleeting instances add up to provide a solid premise for romance.

Mindfulness — The book helps parents be in the present moment for these brief interactions and teaches tools to be able to center themselves when a quick moment arises so that they can truly listen and give their child their undivided attention.

Adaptability – Since no single day is like the other, "5 Minute Parents" offers everyone a timeless measure on how to adopt it for any situation(s) with all age groups.

Education In The Moment: Many routine activities lend themselves to teaching a skill, or at least instilling the love of learning beyond the schoolroom walls.

Emotional Intelligence: It guides the parents and children for developing active awareness about emotions with short exercises and actionable steps.

Practical Application

Parents with careers, single-parents and large families will find "5 Minute Parents" particularly useful. To contemporary parents yearning to make a personal impact in the world but aware of the clock and drawn in so many other directions. But here is the good part: this book offers strategies that are realistic and achievable, useful for someone who feels overwhelmed by normal parenting advice.

Readers will discover: how to establish morning and bedtime rituals, do fast emotional check-ins, and leverage daily activities as opportunities for new lessons. It also teases relationships, tips for communication, conflict resolution, physical touch and mindfulness in just minutes a day.

Finally, "5 Minute Parents" tackles contemporary issues like screen time and how to use technology to bring people together instead of tearing them apart, creative response & responsible screen time through integration, and small actions promote healthy habits.

Conclusion

5 Minute Parents seeks to remind parents about the bigger picture here, celebrating small wins instead of guilt. Consistently and deliberately engaging with kids (even if for a short moment) influences how they grow-up and furthers the family unit.

Welcome to this journey that explores the gems you carry in your pocket everyday behind "5 Minute Parents" and get ready to unlock a world of possibilities. In this inspiring book, you'll learn how to leverage the power of five minutes to create opportunities for growth, connection and joy within your family. So whether you are a brand new parent or have nursed hundreds of little ones through their mischief, this is the parenting book that will change your whole life (and child-rearing) with just one tweak to the way you do things along the way.

Chapter 1

The truth is that today we live in a fast-paced world, where time feels like something unattainable to many of us, and parents often feel stressed out by the everyday needs. The thought of putting in hours into parenting can be intimidating and it almost feels like its an impossible work. But what if I tell you that in just five minutes, you can make a significant impact on your child's life? That's the crux of 5-minute parenting, a philosophy that'll change the way you think about your interactions with your kids in a refreshing way by prioritizing quality over quantity. You can connect with your child and promote their development whilst taking just a few minutes out of your busy day doing so.

Why 5 Minutes Matter

Studies in child psychology suggest that it is less how much time you spend with your children and more the quality of the time spent. Research has shown that the amount of time parents spend with children does not matter too much for their development. It is how parents spend the time they do have that really counts.

How a Few Types of Interactions Matter

Even small, intentional bursts of undivided attention toward our children offer moments that can reverberate in meaningful ways. These short, proactive interactions can strengthen relationships, reinforce a child's self-esteem and provide the emotional support that builds helplessness into health.

Practical and Accessible

Finding five minutes a day for your children is possible, even for the busiest parent. It's about seizing the little opportunities that bubble up naturally over our daily routines. A five-minute conversation on the way to school, a short snuggle before sleep, and a brief joke at breakfast all turn into points of contact with each other.

Maintaining a steady hand and an emotional connection

These short interactions function as anchors over the day, which offer some footing and a sense of security for kids. Research by psychologist John Gottman shows that it is adding up tiny deposits of positive experiences with your child that endear parents and children to each other. They help make kids more resilient, self-confident and socially adept.

The Science Behind It

The social interactions that produce an experience of positivity, even if they are quite brief, release oxytocin — also called the "bonding hormone." It is a hormone that helps us bond and feel safe and trusting. Through repetitive micro-interactions of positivity with our kids, we are reinforcing the parent-child bond over time.

Quality Over Quantity

The 5-minute parenting philosophy is not about swapping for shorter or less meaningful moments, but rather making the most of time we can have with our kids. It's simply about understanding that every minute interaction may change something for you or your child.

Intentional and Mindful

That we use each five minute segment to teach a value, teach something science-y or just show some love. It's about taking advantage of every moment, transforming banal events into incredible moments for connection and development.

Cumulative Effect

Five minutes here and there might not seem like a lot, but multiple instances of five minutes add up over the day and week. The optimal salary only works if small and regular coins of energy.

Being Present

The 5 Minute method teaches parents to be intentional and less negligent with having meaningful moments with the child. Children need this level of presence and this is how their best emotional nourishment happens.

Conclusion

The essence of the 5-minute parenting philosophy is trying to connect with each other no matter how less than ideal the situation or circumstance might be. Especially in our chaotic routines, it is about spreading happiness, lessons and family time. It is a huge step in the direction of not only a better relationship with your child, but also their healthy development as an individual when you embrace this philosophy.

In the next chapter, we will discuss how to make those morning times be great connecting opportunities and transform the often too chaotic AM ritual into functions of bonding and setting a positive tone for the rest of the day.

Chapter 2

With the first light of day peering through window panes a new day starts, filled with examinations to communicate and learn. Phase 1: The Start of Your Day Making Morning Magic After laying down the fast, effective parenting method with the 5-minute parenting philosophy, we now shift focus on what happens at the beginning of each day. Morning rituals, designed with an intentional hand, can help a family to get off on the right foot and set a positive tone which reverberates through warmth into understanding for the rest of the day.

Anyone familiar with the morning rush will recognise an evocative scene from home — parents rushing to get ready for work, kids dashing to be on time for school and a clock that seems to move way too fast. In the midst of this chaos, it may seem like creating purposeful connections is a lost cause. But, oddly enough, this is the time when small intentional acts of connection can do the most for us. Quick breakfast bonding ideas, 5-minute morning pep talks and start-of-the-day habits are brilliant ways for parents to turn the bustling morning into a beloved family ritual.

Quick Breakfast Bonding

Have we all come to the common idea that breakfast is just a mindless duty? It can, however, be painted as a connection. Why not make breakfast together? Parents and children can work together in under five minutes to prepare a healthy smoothie with their favorite fruit, drop them into the blender. When it becomes a time to blend things in the mixer, it turns into moments of braiding conversation together with people as we exchange delicious nuggets about each other. That tiny moment of coming together makes for a solid healthy start to the day and the gentle reminder that family is there to support, nurture, and rely on each other.

Another idea to bond is setting up a rotating "treat breakfast". Every day, one family member gets to choose what is for breakfast (within reason). It keeps things fun, and also shows kids to be mindful of what other people would like versus not want, and how everyone can enjoy an occasional treat. Those conversations, however short, pave the way for children to talk about what they like or dislike and get validation from parents.

5-Minute Morning Pep Talks

This ends the more practical part of breakfast, and starts the emotional journey with 5-minute morning pep talks. These short, intentional talks are reminders of positivity that keep parents and children grounded. A good morning pep talk is brief, and specific. Instead of generic encouragements, think about the specific challenges or promises of opportunity that the day may hold.

For example, if your child has a school presentation to give, you might pep talk them by asking one thing about the presentation that they are excited for and one thing they are nervous for. A brief check-in like this acknowledges the child's feelings, provides an opportunity for targeted support and helps put the upcoming event in proper perspective. But being nervous is normal and telling a personal story about how you got through the fear helps further promote that bravery is not a lack of fear, but coming back to who you are despite it.

As child psychologist Dr. Elena Martinez puts it, "Just a few minutes of undivided positive attention in the morning acts as an inoculation against potential stresses they might experience throughout the day. It's like arming them with emotional armor." And it is these simple moments that may end up shaping a child most, their emotional resilience and wellbeing.

Positive Start-of-Day Habits

Another important thing to do is build positive habits at the beginning of your day. Their habits become the bones on which children base their approach to daily life. One of the habits is a "gratitude minute" where each family member says something they are grateful for. This cultivates a culture of optimism and trains all to habitually search for the positive in their lives.

The next one is really strong: "Intention setting." Family members take turns in one or two minutes stating their primary goal or intention for the day. This ten minute exercise has the benefit of giving children focus and a sense of purpose which may otherwise be missing in an unstructured holiday. But when parents model this behavior, the children learn to prioritize and set goals.

Something else that can be done in the morning that seems to also make a huge difference is including physical movement into it. Just a couple of minutes to shake your booty while dressing up or doing some stretches can wake up bodies and minds. These are healthy things that add a little bit of fun to lining kids up in routine, and help wash away the crankiness.

Conclusion

And when it comes to morning rituals for connection, the takeaway is less about perfection and more about consistency & intention. Not every morning they will be responsive and not every conversation with them will hit the deep. But by doing these little bits of bonding at breakfast, 5-minute pep talks as they get to the car and being a Good Morning habit starter when around, parents can create a ripple effect of reassurance that extends through the day and beyond.

Nevertheless, these morning rituals are great weapons in the 5-minute parent's arsenal: even in a busy household, they provide an opportunity for meaningful interactions. Next we will take a look at how you can use these principles for other moments in your child's day, especially bedtime bonding. The morning habits and relationships provide the foundation of a gentle, loving environment that envelopes the family as it wraps itself up at the end of each day.

Chapter 3

As the morning turns to day and then evening, moms and dads found it tough to lift their kids out of daytime vibrance into nighttime oasis. Known colloquially as the "witching hour," this important time can quickly become fraught. That being said, it does provide an incredibly great opportunity to connect in a meaningful way through abbreviated bedtime traditions. With the 5 minutes parenting model, parents can change these moments to be meaningful, where we build connections and make memories. Imagine snuggling in the evening to listen to a calm story or have shared silence—these mini-rituals not only provide assurance and warmth but also a happy context in their minds for when they fall asleep.

Bedtime routines are more than just a way to get kids to sleep, they are the perfect opportunity for connection and development. Dr. Laura Markham, clinical psychologist and parenting expert at Aha! Parenting says of this time: "The last experience your child has before going to sleep will set the tone for his night (and often yours) as well as for that next day." And this really highlights how important it is to use the last moments before sleep — however short they may be,

Bedtime Routines that Have Real Substance

These short but significant bedtime routines send a message to the child's body and mind that it is time to unwind from the day, builds predictability and safety, while creating intentional connection. The trick is to do this in small doses and through the 5-minute rule, which is a principled value that argues helping your employees exercise their spirits by engaging with you only for brief amounts of time makes quite an impression.

Simple but effective, this might involve taking a quick bath or washing up as well, freshening into pajamas, brushing teeth and ending in bed together with your little one to hear a short story or talk quietly. Each step has the possibility of connection infused within. As an example, while brushing your child's teeth, a "tooth-brushing dance" is appropriate or a short song about creating healthy oral care habits could be sung to make the task fun and establish oral hygiene routines.

The Magic of Storytelling

But when it is time to get into bed, that is where the storytelling part comes and the real bonding starts. Quick storytelling techniques are a highly fruitful approach that creates an inviting and homey environment as well to inspire his imagination and language abilities. One option is called the Three-Sentence Story — parents begin a story in one sentence, then the child continues with the second sentence then finishes off in the third. Completions: This collaborative storytelling fits within the 5-minute timeframe and drives creativity while developing narrative skills.

The next is also a fun way to do it called the 'Story in a Jar' Write suggestions or use small things and fill a jar by both parents and children. Every night one item is pulled and a mini story is made around it. This keeps storytelling fresh and interesting, while also training kids to think on their feet and create stories from simple cues—all in a matter of minutes.

If parents don't feel particularly confident in their ability to tell a story, short illustrated books that are meant to be read quickly at bedtime work tremendously well. There are many collections of "5-minute stories" from publishers with whole, engaging stories ideal for this. They tell a good story and do not make bedtime last an age.

Reflections on the Day / List of Thanks

This is another great time to do your nightly reflections or gratitude. Doing this helps create a positive mindset and aid them process their day, helping them set up for slumber. One of my favorite exercises is called, Three Good Things that have a round parent and child tell about three positive experiences they had during the day. You may do this in as little as two or three moments, however it carries deep impacts on the health and fitness of both baby and parent.

In his groundbreaking research on positive psychology, Dr. Martin Seligman discovered that expressing gratitude this way can have powerful effects of enhancing mood and increasing life satisfaction. According to him: "Gratitude improves the quality of your life and increases the amount of happiness. In the moment when we feel grateful, we are taking advantage of a pleasant recollection from our life. Including this 2-minute practice in the evening helps promote a mindset of positive thinking and reflection as a daily habit for children.

The "Worry Drop" Technique

A second one that is also brief but powerful at bedtime with kids is called the Worry Drop. This includes a red box or jar that kids can "put" worries in before going to sleep. The child lists out their worries, writes and/or draws them on a small paper, then drops it in the container. This small action helps ease anxiety and provides a feeling of relief, making sleep easier.

The Power of Physical Touch

One of the key components of bedtime bonding that can be included in short routines is physical touch. We know that touch allows us to connect with one another as human beings; several studies prove it promotes reduced stress, improved immune function and creates a sensation of safety. A distracting and playful back rub, soft head massage or just holding hands while talking makes the emotional impact of this part of her daily routine amazing.

"Touch is ten times more powerful than a word or an emotion, it reaches us all the time," Dr. Tiffany Field, director of the Touch Research Institute at the University of Miami School of Medicine adds. Except, touch arouses you like no other sense." A quick 30-second back rub will release oxytocin (the so-called "bonding hormone") and help facilitate a feeling of closeness between parent and child.

Consistency is Key

Well as this window into bonding time before bed draws to a close let us not forget; consistency is everything. Each part of the routine individually takes a few minutes, but over time they compound. Through these bedtime rituals that embody brevity and significance, parents can cultivate a nightly wellspring of connection in the face of busy lives.

These 5-minute bedtime bonding techniques are so simple and flexible. They can be designed according to the individual preferences and requirements of each family and may also evolve over time with children as they grow and their interests change. So what stays the same are the messages these rituals convey: that there is always time for connection, love and care even on days when it gets hectic.

In moving to the following section on emotional check-ins, we will dive into how these principles of brief and intentional interactions throughout the day can help develop greater emotional intelligence and allow for a safe space to express. Although the bedtime routine is such a significant bookend to the day, it must be emphasized that there are many more opportunities for meaningful connections throughout our daily lives.

Chapter 4

Last chapter was all about this time together at bedtime. As we move onto the next, remember that emotional well-being is the foundation of today's child's development. In this chapter you will learn how periodic, purposeful emotional check-ins can dramatically present a boost to your child with regards to their emotional intelligence and with regards to your relationship with them.

Emotions are the unseen currents that flow through everything we experience, tinting and giving texture to our lives. Having the emotional support of an adult who has lived through many feelings can be a true beacon for children, who are not quite ready to navigate that map themselves. And as parents we have the best chance to be that guide, even amongst the busiest of days. Emotional check-ins are quick but effective: in five minutes, we can offer our children an emotional safe place to play around with their feelings.

Think of icebreaker exercises for emotional intelligence

First, Allow us to explore what short stints of emotional intelligence exercises are. Emotional intelligence (or EQ) refers to the ability to identify and understand our own emotions, as well as being able to identify, understand and influence the feelings of others. A high EQ will help children to create good relationships, have better mental health, and be more successful in school and life. The positive side is that emotional intelligence can be cultivated and honed, with low-impact interactions spread over time — rather than the traditional model of intensive training one-off sessions.

A good activity is to use the "Emotion Wheel," which is a simple and effective exercise. Make a big colored wheel that is split into sections to show different emotions. In your five-minute check-in, have the child point to the emotion they are experiencing. This helps them not only figure out how they feel but also grow their emotional vocabulary. As psychologist Dr. John Gottman writes, "Emotion coaching begins with the parent's awareness of the child's emotions." When we teach our children to name their feelings, we are helping them take a first step in making sense of and managing those emotions.

An even faster exercise is the "Body Scan". Lead your child in a short body scan, encouraging them to observe any physical symptoms of their emotions. For example, they might feel some tightness in their chest when they're nervous or warmth in their cheeks when they're happy. It can help children be more aware of their feelings and lay the groundwork for future stress management skills.

Quick approaches to handle sensations

Next, quick tips on dealing with feelings: Remember that you can NOT fix or change your child's emotion — only validate it. An example of this is a technique by Dr. Dan Siegel called "Name it to Tame it." Identifying it often lessens the blow when a child is really struggling with an emotion. For instance: "Sounds like you are feeling frustrated at the moment. Is that right?" Just naming the emotion activates the prefrontal cortex – our place of rational thought – and calms the emotional limbic system.

An additional quick strategy we would like to share is the "Feelings Thermometer." Similar to how a thermometer works, draw one for your little and have them show you where they feel on the scale. This is a beautiful visual that can assist the child who has difficulty with words and gets that feeling from a quick picture of how strong this feeling is. From there, you can respond with comfort, problem solving or just listen.

Provide a safe environment to express

Possibly one of the most important things about emotional check-ins, creating a safe space for expression in just a few minutes. Kids need to know that all feelings are okay, including the hard ones. The Emotion Box activity is one way you can create this safe space. How about giving your child a little box or jar to write or draw their feelings and put them inside? If your child would like to go over these, you may do so during your check-in time. That gets out physical feelings but also shows you are aware and care about their feelings.

According to Dr. John Gottman, who did extensive research on emotional safety, "in an emotionally safe environment children discover that their feelings matter—that it is all right to express them—and that their parents will support them in coping with difficult emotions." It takes only a few minutes a day to cultivate this form of safety, in which no elaborate defenses need to be established or anything long-winded explained — just the routine and its inherent acceptance.

A second fast way to cultivate that emotional safety is with the use of I-statements. Remind your child to use "I feel" statements This allows them to own their emotions and minimizes blame or defensiveness in conversations. For example, instead of "You never listen to me," they may say, "I feel ignored when I am not heard." This tiny tweak in vernacular makes an enormous difference inside the household when it comes to experiencing or communicating with feelings.

And keep in mind, this is not only about what we say but about the way we communicate without using words when creating a safe space for sharing feelings. And during these brief moments of an emotional check-in, have eye contact, sound sweet in your voice and give a pat on the back if suitable. These subtle signals can communicate a lot about your openness and acceptance of where your child is emotionally.

The Benefits for Parents

Now that we are nearing the end of this session, remember emotional check-ins are not only great for your child but for you as a parent too. These mini sessions offer glimpses into your child's universe and help you navigate through their fears, needs and joys better. Not only are you modeling emotional awareness and expression, but you're also providing your child with some of the most important life skills they'll need as they grow into their own independence.

As Dr. Marc Brackett, author of the book Permission to Feel, eloquently states: "When we are able to recognize, understand, label, express and regulate our emotions — the skills we call emotional intelligence — our emotions can serve as important sources of information for how we think and behave... Emotions provide a compass to motivate us in our decisions and interactions with others ... they play a major role in shaping the quality of our physical health as well as the success of our relationships."

Conclusion

To recap our conversation on emotional check-ins, consistency is your best friend. Practicing these five-minute interactions regularly will set a good emotional foundation for your child. These are ways that create daily space for connection, understanding and growth. The following chapter will explore how we can shift these moments into learning opportunities, by leveraging the emotions awareness developed here to unlock curiosity and cognitive growth.

Chapter 5

Now, moving away from the emotional parts we've touched upon, here is something you could do towards your child's intellectual side. This chapter will show you how to create lessons from day-to-day experiences in five minutes. Micro-learning is designed in a way that it does not feel like one other activity that one needs to do, rather, it feels integrated into daily life and things become natural.

Making Everyday Scenarios a Chance to Learn

But parents who turn the most mundane of daily tasks into learning moments are masters of their craft. Take something simple like separating the laundry. For young children, this basic chore can be a colorful lesson in colors, shapes and sorting. While folding clothes, use the opportunity to talk about colors with your child. Check out this red number nerd robe! What do you see that is red in this pile? Both of these help you identify colors as well as focus and enhance language skills by repeating them out loud.

Laundry sorting can also take the form of a math lesson for older children. "We have 10 socks in total. How many full pairs do we have if we pair them up? These are necessary for cleaning and keeping your house tidy, which this quick exercise helps with introducing basic division and pairs. And the secret is to make all of this require that you see every day a thing with an aspect of education.

Cooking Up Learning

Preparing a meal is also another treasure trove of little micro-learning moments. Cooking requires measurement, following instructions and great wisdom about cause and effect — all valuable skills for children. If you are running short of time, still there are small ways in which you can engage your kid and make learning a big outcome. Let your child do the measuring when preparing pancakes, for example; if you are making pancakes, let them measure out the flour. It also introduces volume and shows how precise you must be when following a recipe.

Talk through the process as you cook and ask questions to get your child thinking critically. Question: "If I add blue food coloring, and then yellow food color, what do you think will happen?" This quick activity gives a lesson on color theory and predicts something—that is some essential science skills. Getting kids into the kitchen with you is not only teaching them about making food, but also providing the foundation for chemistry, math and following multi-step directions.

Grocery Store Adventures

A simple trip to the grocery store can become a new opportunity for learning. As you are shopping, turn it into a challenge for your child to identify an example of each shape. "Where can you find something round in this aisle?" This game utilizes sharpened observation and refines geometry concepts. Older children can practice math skills comparing prices and calculating discounts. E. If this cereal is 20% off the regular price of $5, what will it sell for? These quick calculations sharpen math skills and show real-world uses for arithmetic.

Nature Walk Discoveries

Nature walks, no matter how short, are full of learning moments. Teach your child to observe and ask questions while observing the things around him/her. Why are you changing the color to some leaves? With just this single question, you can talk about seasons, photosynthesis and life cycles! A five-minute walk becomes a biology and environmental science lesson, in which students learn that the act of observation takes practice.

Car Ride Games

One another often-missed micro-learning moment is the car ride to school or activities. Engage in word games that build vocabulary and develop language skills. For example, a twist on the classic "I Spy" game is to make it letter sound-based: "I spy something that begins with the /b/ b/ sound." Not only does this occupy time, but it also supports phonemic awareness, which is an important reading component.

Audiobooks are awesome tools for learning when traveling a little further. If you read between the lines, select a book just above your child's reading level and have an informal discussion afterward! By reading high-quality books, they are exposed to enriching vocabulary and idiomatic sentence structures, building language skills passively. Additionally, it instills a passion for narrative and literacy that pays dividends in the classroom later.

Quick Educational Games

Short, 5-minute educational games and activities are a secret weapon in your learning tool belt as a parent. The trick is to have a selection of fast, fun games you can pull out at the drop of a hat. So one of those is Categories. Pick a category—animals, for instance—and take turns naming as many as you can in one-minute intervals. It promotes recalling, extends knowledge and can be applied to almost any subject area.

A very fast but efficient game: "What Is Missing?" Place a few items on a tray, let your child look at them for a few seconds and then take one object away while they close their eyes. This game hones the attention to detail and memory. For bigger kids you could use more items, or tougher objects so that it stays a challenge.

Quick-fire games give you the opportunity to practice math facts. Number Bonds Number bonds are a fast method of making addition and subtraction sticks. Say a number and ask your child to say 2 numbers that add to it. So if you say 10 they may answer 7 and three or 6 and four. This will help children in developing mental math and understanding the relationship between numbers.

If your goal for using the internet is to improve vocabulary and spelling, then word-building games are a fantastic option. It is a short game where you have to create words by changing one letter at a time (such as 'Word Ladder'). For example change from cat, to bat, then bet, then bee. Game- This is a game that will help to expand vocabulary while providing an opportunity to learn word patterns and spelling rules.

Cultivating Curiosity

Micro-learning moments, by far the most precious of their type, are places where we become curious in small amounts. Therefore, the aim is not only to teach but also to inspire a lifelong love for learning. It starts with you modeling curiosity yourself. Why not expose your surprise and curiosity out loud when you see something strange? "Wow, I've never seen a flower like that!" I wonder what it's called?" This shows that learning never stops and there is nothing wrong in not knowing some facts.

Help your child to be curious, and have lots of questions, however stupid it may sound. As the physicist Richard Feynman said, I would rather have questions that can't be answered than answers that can't be questioned. This disposition to learning—prioritizing inquiry above memorization—is what cultivates the conditions for higher thinking.

If your child ever asks something you just absolutely cannot answer, make a point to model how research is done. "That's a great question! Let's look it up together." And even if you might spend a few minutes or more looking for the answer, you are opening the mind of your child to learn how to look for information by themselves and that is what matters in an era where knowledge is everything.

Wonder Moments

Yes, I really would love to see some of this — wonder moments built into your everyday life. During dinner, invite each family member to share what they learned or were wondering about that day. This not only reinforces that Learning is continuous but also promotes reflection and verbalisation of thought which are important cognitive skills.

Conclusion

These micro-learning moments are not intended to add pressure or force every conversation into a semi-formal lesson. Rather, it is focused on creating a culture of learning that will happen organically, naturally, and with joy over the long run. When we look for teachable moments in everyday situations – we show our kids that education is not just limited to the classroom.

In summation, micro-learning moments are brief interactions that have the potential to substantially impact a child's brain growth. Those five-minute learning opportunities, woven into everyday life, form the basis for a lifelong journey of exploration and discovery. The next chapter, however, is about an equally important skill of parenting — the art of listening. We will learn that attending fully, even for a brief period of time, may really change the way we communicate with our kids and expand our ability to comprehend their requirements and perspectives.

Chapter 6

Now, transitioning from the micro-learning moments covered in the previous chapter to a crucial tool that can greatly boost our parenting effectiveness, I wish to discuss active listening. In this age of fast-food with distractions aplenty and no time for listening (or so we say) the skill of genuinely listening to our children has never been needed more. In this chapter, we are going to discover how we can play the game of being in the moment, how non-verbal communication plays an essential part in our overall communication skills and few exercises which would take no more than 5 minutes to help you hear better all while keeping it practical with our 5-minute parenting philosophy.

Being able to transpose Sense of Urgency into How To Focus

Prioritized attention is the foundation of active listening. We need to not just hear what our kids say but be part of their thoughts, their feelings and experiences. This skill is even more important with 5-minute parenting. These moments of connection are often fleeting, and we need to find a way to ensure our children feel listened to too.

Another great practice for this focused listening is the full-body listen. This means your whole body reflects engagement. If your kid comes up to talk, stop completely. Eye contact, lean in a little, body out. That shift in space lets your child know that they have your full attention (even if just for a few minutes).

Dre. Adele Faber, who co-wrote How to Talk So Kids Will Listen & Listen So Kids Will Talk and over a dozen other classic parenting books, emphasizes that "This is so powerful because when we listen with our undivided attention (and without interjecting the tentacles of our own story), we're communicating to them that they matter. I care what you have to say.' Telling their child that they are proud of them can go a long way in building self-esteem and openness in communication with your little one.

The other important factor in focused attention is being present mentally. Our minds can easily drift away — even when we are physically present — in this multitasking world. When involving your child, practice discovering a means to empty out your mind of other thoughts. It's ok if your mind wonders, but then try to focus back on now – what is your child saying. It takes practice but this mental discipline can immediately improve your interactions.

If you're doing your 5-minutes of listening, try applying the "do not interrupt" rule. Do not jump in when your child is talking to provide your guidance, insist on the correctness of something they said, or tell them about a similar thing you had done in the past. Instead, absorb what they are saying. This does not mean that you cannot respond at all, but the responses should be directed towards eliciting further expression. Responses such as "I see," "Tell me more," or even that sounds interesting are simple ways to keep the conversation going without redirecting it.

Understanding Non-Verbal Cues

Much of our communication is non-verbal. Some research says non-verbal cues account for 93% of effective communication. As parents owning and tuning into what those cues look like can vastly increase our ability to relate to our children.

One of the most noticeable types of non-verbal communication is through facial expressions. A furrowed brow followed by a slight frown or, better yet, a shining smile can say tons about how your child feels. Listen carefully to these subtle signs in your conversations — they often point towards emotions that are beyond the written or spoken word for your child.

Yet another important factor is body language. Observe the way your kid is standing or sitting. Do they have a hunchback indicating an allergic reaction, or discomfort and insecurity? Or are they sitting upright, almost like little soldiers—we think of it as a confident or excited posture? These physical signals add context to the words and reinforces all of the communication actually happening.

But also, being mindful of your own demeanor. Children are also better listeners than we think and can read some of our subtle signs. It means keeping your arms and legs uncrossed. Acknowledge that you are listening by nodding. You can also create empathy and connection by mirroring your child's face.

The tone of your voice is another non-verbal signal that it carries much weight. Not just what we say, but the manner of our speech. Notice how your child's words come out: the pitch, volume, and cadence. An uncertain note may suggest a fear, while vehement, fitful delivery again may express exuberance — or a rage. Listening to these vocal cues gives you insights into your child's mood, and a chance to respond effectively.

Dr. John Gottman, world expert on relationships, describes parent child interactions as requiring emotional attunement. Identifying feelings in a child means observing the way they move and what they're doing with their face, as well as their tone of voice, and even something along the lines of what's happening around them, according to him. You can take 5 minutes to offer this attunement and it will move your relationship with a child closer together.

Listening Exercise in 5 minutes

Now, how about a couple of short exercises to work on your listening? Enjoying these can be added to your routine, and all take a few minutes each day needed to practice on making you an active listener.

The "repeat back" technique is a strong exercise. End your child's speech by summarizing what they are saying in your own words. Not only does this prove that you are actually listening, it gives your child a chance to clear up any confusion. For instance: "So if I am getting this right you are upset that your friend did not invite you to play in the game during recess. Is that right?" It also honors the emotions your child may be experiencing and allows you both to communicate clearly about the situation going on, showing them that you hear what they are saying.

The second helpful exercise is the "emotion labeling" practice. When you hear your child, listen and identify the feelings they are stating. For example, you might say something like "It sounds like you're disappointed," or "I can hear the excitement in your voice." Consequently, your child develops emotional literacy through this concept of common ground and feels seen in more than just a physical sense.

One is called "curiosity questions," where you ask your child open-ended questions that show you're interested in what they think and went through. Ask questions starting with What, How or Tell me about instead of yes/no type questions. Something like, "What was your favorite part of today." or "How did it make you feel when that happened?" These questions promote longer and more detailed answers and indicate to your child that you are actually interested in what they have to say.

A great example of this is the "daily download" exercise — and you only need five minutes to do it. Give your child five minutes each day of uninterrupted talk time where they can talk about anything, without you judging them or telling them how wrong they are. Maybe it is at bedtime, or during the drive home from school, or any other consistent time that fits into your family schedule. The trick is to create this as routine, a safe space for honest and open dialogue.

Dr. Laura Markham, clinical psychologist and parenting expert, recommends this kind of listening time. If children feel heard, they are more likely to listen to and cooperate with their parents, she said. Trust is earned and trust is not built in a moment. Trust takes time only to be focused on regularity."

Conclusion

These are things we need to practice; these techniques, as any skill you develop will get better the more you do it. While you may not have constant hours to constantly discuss things with your child, these 5-minute conversations will establish a practice of communication in your household.

Active listening is not merely to extract information, but to connect, trust and comprehend. If your children know that they are really listened to, they will bring their problems to you; everyday happiness and will look for advice from you. At its core, active listening is all about removing those barriers to creating a lasting parent-child bond.

With this chapter about the different ways to practice active listening, we transition smoothly into our next subject — the theme of praise and encouragement. The skills we've covered in this post—concentration, observation of non-verbal communication, and more intentional listening exercises—will provide tools as we dive into strategies for increasing how to praise children and elevate their self-esteem through appropriate reaffirmation. So to create this positive space for listening and discussing our values as a family — which is what serves best ahead of time when it comes real — together with following our 5-minute parenting with active listening (and lots of funny sound effects), then we are building the growth situation.

Chapter 7

This next dimension of parenting–prior to the methods of praise and encouragement from Chapter 3: — transitions from the active listening techniques discussed previously, and with movement forward in this manner comes another much needed ability we must cultivate. Listening is the first step in understanding our children, but praise and encouragement build on listening to give them self-confidence and motivation to grow as learners.

How Specific, Timely Praise Can Transform People

Specific, timely praise is so powerful! Praise that is specific – rather than generically given – points to certain actions or characteristics, reinforcing what we want them to repeat and also enhancing a child's sense of competence. When delivered with specific details and in a timely manner, praise is one of the most effective means we have to influence students' behavior and self-image.

Think about the difference between "That was great" and "I saw how you stacked those blocks carefully together to build such a tall tower. Took some patience there and experienced hands!" The latter not only celebrates the child's success but also affirms effort and skill. This specificity allows children to know precisely what they are doing right, so they repeat those behaviors.

Timing is equally crucial. When praise is given as soon as possible after a child does something good, the two are associated in your child's mind. So, for example, if a child helps set the table to have dinner together and you praise them right after that it will mean much more than praising them hours or the next day.

Balancing Praise

Praise is a powerful tool but should be used judiciously. But, if you overdo it or praise for the wrong things, it can backfire. Children are all-controlling and easily recognize when they get compliments with any little ounce of authenticity or exaggeration. It can create distrust in future compliments or become dependent on others to tell them their work is worthy as a means of gauging their own worth. You need to be the one that by receiving so much recognition will become a trophy for being genuine and comparable, Real Work, while trophies are awarded in exceptional circumstances. It will help children to develop real confidence and feel grounded within themselves by letting them know what they have really achieved.

5-Minute Recognition Rituals

Having a 5-minute recognition ritual in a day can immensely change the parent-child relationship and helps elevate confidence and motivation levels for children. These short but impactful moments can take many forms and can be integrated into the flow of your family life.

For instance, during dinner time you might implement a "proudest moment" practice where everyone in the household shares something they were proud of that day. This prompts reflection on their performance and offers a chance to give praise that is detailed and relevant.

It could be a nice bedtime ritual — an "appreciation moment" at the end of your day to take 5 minutes. When you go to tuck in your child, take a moment to highlight something specific that you appreciated about their behavior or effort that day. Ending the day positively is a great way to affirm good behaviors and send your child off to sleep with positivity, feeling appreciated and loved.

For preschool age children, a praise chart can be especially effective. Set up a "star chart" or "recognition board," where you can ready stickers or notes to quickly recognize certain positive behaviors during the course of an ongoing day. Having them see their accomplishments like this can be very motivating and also a reminder of who they are and how far they have really come.

Using Affirmations As A Way To Create Self Esteem

Another effective strategy, like the whole 5-minute parenting method is to build self-esteem through bite-sized affirmations. Self-esteem does not happen overnight, it is the culmination of positive reinforcement and success. Even just short, periodic affirmations can go a long way toward this.

Recognize your kid's strengths and positive traits that you've seen – kindness, creativity, perseverance, curiosity (the list goes on.) After that, write down some short and specific affirmations for these qualities. Such as, "You are so kind and considerate to others" or "Your creativity never ceases to amaze me." Recite these affirmations to your child often, incorporating them into your morning or bedtime rituals.

Just as important is that they are honest and based on what you actually observed. Children are aware of inauthenticity and insincere praise can cause more harm than a complete lack of praise. We want to reinforce these healthy, positive beliefs about themselves as we do not want them dependent on us feeding their ego.

Promoting Process instead of Product

However, true self-confidence is built by praising effort instead of just results. Do not just praise the results; Praise the process Reinforce process, not outcome — Rather than making a good grade the end goal, praise the effort and study behavior that got you there. An approach like this encourages a growth mindset in children, encouraging them to understand that their abilities can be cultivated over time with effort and perseverance.

Be intentional with your language as you use these praise and encouragement strategies. Do not make comparisons where your child is concerned. Telling your child things like, "You are the most brilliant one in class" or "You are way smarter than your brother," can eventually lead to pressure and make room for unhealthy competition. Rather, stand by who your child is and the things they accomplish.

Also, be careful not to use praise as a manipulation tool. To be clear, we all want to assertively encourage some behaviors and not others, but using praise simply as a means to an end can backfire. Kids can initiate doing things simply to gain praise instead of developing their internal motivation. We want children to feel good about themselves and their efforts, not as if they need validation from others to foster a behavior reliant on this phenomenon. We are instead directing them to a sense of internal pride in their efforts and achievements as well as healthy self-esteem for life!

More Than Just Academics or Sports

And these words should not be just for academic or sports success. Acknowledge and reinforce positive character traits, kindness, problem-solving abilities, and empathy. This full-fledged method to praise assists kids nurture a wholesome self-worth which doesn't simply rely upon achievements that they obtain externally.

Just keep in mind that the way we talk about achievement to our children can have ripple effects on how long those apples will stay on your tree. As psychologist Carol Dweck has stated, "Praising children's intelligence harms their motivation and it harms their performance." She is instead a proponent of providing praise based on effort, strategy and process. Bottom line, it creates resilience and a love of learning, not a fear of failure or fixed mindset about ability.

Conclusion

The good news is that using these praise and encouragement techniques takes very little time. What I love most about the 5-minute parenting approach, is that these special and impactful ways of connecting can be infused into your everyday life. A few words of encouragement before school, acknowledging a nice thing he/she did that day, or celebrating any small win— these little things can leave a huge mark on your child during their formative years.

In closing this chapter on praise and encouragement, it's evident that these seemingly minor moments are important due to their impact on our child's self-worth and drive. Providing specific praise, timely recognition and authentic affirmation creates an atmosphere of positivity and encourages confidence.

The next chapter will be on conflict resolution, and after creating a framework of positive reinforcement, the power of praise and encouragement to help build their self-esteem so we can work through the disasters family life brings. They can be invaluable tools for constructive praise, building self-worth, learning how to overcome differences and creating problem solving skills in the little time windows that our busy lives allow.

Chapter 8

Moving on from the last chapter of praise and encouragement, we must keep in mind that no matter how good a relationship is between the parent-child conflicts will inevitably occur. It's not about eliminating conflict, but rather minimizing it and the negative impact it has on overall productivity. This chapter talks about how parents can be done fighting their child in under 5 minutes, while teaching vital life skills.

Fast Strategies for Making a Situation Less Difficult

Generally, step one amid rising emotions is to lower the temperature. A simple approach is the "pause and breathe" technique. Take three deep breaths together (great practice for you and your child) before continuing the discussion. This one simple act can provide a brief mental pause, an opportunity for everyone to take a breath and regroup. Dr. Daniel Siegel, clinical professor of psychiatry at the UCLA School of Medicine, writes "When we pause then we are much more likely to respond and not react."

The other quick de-escalation strategy is the change of scenery. If things get heated in one part of the house, recommend going to another room or even going outside for a minute. The change in your physical state can trigger a mental one and give you an objective view of what is happening. The family is a microcosm. — Virginia Satir If we think about family, where the married couple lives with their children, it quickly becomes clear that there are many different kinds of marriage and families around the world! You can change the entire society if you change your functioning inside the family.

Structured Problem Solving Is Best Taught in Short Bursts

SADAS: a powerful five-minute lesson in problem-solving. SODAS – Situation, Options, Disadvantages and Advantages and Solution Begin with a clear statement of the problem. Next, list three possible approaches that you may use to tackle it. Briefly discuss the pros and cons of each option. Then collaboratively select the best solution.

So, if the conflict is homework not being done, it may look like this: "Math homework isn't finished and it's almost time for bed." Those choices might be to work through the night, work up early to have it done before class or imperfect. Rapidly consider the relative merits and hazards of each, then come to a joint conclusion about the best way forward. This not only addresses the immediate issue but also teaches critical thinking and decision-making abilities.

Quick Reconciliation Techniques

A concept with hidden strength is the "I feel" sentence. To help your child use feelings, teach them to express them with the line: "I feel [emotion] when [situation] because [reason]. For example: "When you take my toys without asking, I feel upset because I was still using them." This technique allows kids to express how they are feeling without saying it in a way that is blaming or attacking, and breaks the barrier for more productive conversation.

This is a variation of the quick reconciliation method called "apology and amends". So, require a true apology accompanied by a clear step that attempts to right the wrong. It could simply be giving a hug, assisting with chores, or drawing a little. The trick is to not just apologize, but to show some kind of remorse and a will (and deed) to reconcile.

Another tool is the "agreement for next time". Once you have dealt with the present situation, spend a minute on approach to avoiding similar conflicts down the road. This paradigm encourages children to learn from their blunders and be equipped with problem-solving skills. If your issue was a misunderstanding around chores, you could agree to make an easily vi-as-able chore chart for future reference.

The Role of Humor

Expectation versus reality: The role of humor in the rapid resolution of conflict A perfectly placed joke, joking facial expression even will sometimes temper and at least knock down the tension to a level where creativity can enter now as well. But remember that humor should never become a tool to mask, undermine or undermine your child. Author and educator Adele Faber says "Humor is one of the best ways to diffuse a situation, but never at the expense of your child's feelings."

The Agreement Jar

A different fast way for dealing with repeated fights is the "agreement jar". Have an empty jar and small bit of paper ready Whenever you and your child have worked out a plan for how they will handle a particular situation, write it down and add it to the jar. You can pull these solutions out in future fights, wasting less time and avoiding bigger headaches.

Teaching Compromise

Compromise is a must when it comes to dealing with conflicts, and teaching your children how to do this is incredibly important. A leading method for achieving common ground is the "meet in the middle" approach. When there is a conflict over screen time for example begin with each stating what you would like the ideal to be. Next, compromise and meet each other halfway to somewhat satisfy both parties. This way, we both not only solve the immediate conflict but also learn how to negotiate.

Conclusion

Keep in mind that the intention of these rapid conflict resolution strategies is not merely to stop disagreements, but rather promote understanding, strengthen relationships, and help equip your child with necessary life skills. With practice, you might notice that conflicts are less common and intense. Your chant will redefine your home to a place where arguments are not something that is seen as a problem but rather an avenue for you to grow and learn.

Be prepared to practice these techniques and be patient as you begin using them — don;t get too bummed out if they don't go perfectly immediately! Conflict resolution is the kind of skill that gets better with time and lots of practice. In the next chapter, we'll see how short dips of warmth and physical affection can enhance your connection with your child to support the communication skills presented here.

Chapter 9

Transitioning from conflict resolution, another area that always has an affective component is physical contact and affection. In this chapter briefly connecting a morsel of physical compassion that can change the micro-moments in a fifty-year-old half of second will effectively move into the circle of intimacy levels family contains.

The Importance of Tangible Bonds

In this fast-paced world of ours, with everyone glued to their phones and on social media via digital interaction, a simple touch can make all the difference. According to Director Tiffany Field of the Touch Research Institute at the University of Miami School of Medicine, "Touch is ten times more powerful than verbal or emotional contact and it has a strong impact on almost everything we do. Touch — or even just the thought of it — can arouse you like no other sense. Our kids — and our connection with them — is affected by the simplest physical contact.

The Benefits of Touch

Touch is the primary need of all human beings — and children even more so. Necessary for healthy growth and emotional development Touch, whether from a child or another adult, seems to be good for us physically — reducing stress hormones and increasing the so-called bonding hormone known as oxytocin, along with some markers of immune function. This will lead to benefits that go well beyond infancy to children of all ages, including teenagers.

Your 5-minute parent philosophy: It is not the time spent that matters, it is the quality of this time. Short, deliberate touches can be powerful. A hug before school, a warm stroke on the back during homework, or a high five after a task—we can use simple actions that speak volumes of love, support and encouragement to our children.

The Power of a Hug

The hug is one of the most potent physical contact ways that is short. Even a brief hug can transmit safety, comfort, and unconditional love. According to neuroscientist Dr. Paul Zak, long hugs for 20 seconds or longer can cause the release of oxytocin which can increase bonding between two persons and decrease levels of stress. You may not always be able to fit in a 20-second hug, but shorter hugs can still bring plenty of benefits. Consider establishing a "morning hug" to make it part of the routine—before school, get in a quick squeeze; it does wonders for setting up a good day and serves as an emotional glue.

High-Fives and Gentle Touches

For older kids and teens who aren't into hugs, a quick high-five is also a good way to sneak in some brief physical contact. A high five can be to acknowledge an achievement, a booster of encouragement or just tell your child you see them. It's a short but mighty message to say, "I'm proud of you, I see you. Giving high-fives when your child does something you want to encourage, tries hard to work on a task, or just walks by often provides many brief instances which allow encouragement throughout the day.

A soothing touch like a hand upon the arm or a pat on the back does wonders too. These light touches can offer support, comfort, and company without being overwhelming. But when your kid gets stuck on their homework, a hand on their arm and words of encouragement can offer emotional support and an anchor in the moment. Likewise, a gentle rub when your son or daughter is feeling blue can communicate more empathy and concern than verbalizing that love.

Using the Touch You Have In Your Daily Life

Integrating touch into everyday life ensures that you get regular physical contact with your child. And bedtime rituals are a great time to do this. A kiss goodnight, a soft rub on the back or even just a 3-minute foot massage can ease your child into a feeling of comfort and security before falling asleep. These night-time touches are a reassurance and bedtime becomes associated with positive feelings which makes it easier for the baby to fall asleep without worrying about bedtime as a way of being our eldest child.

Touching toddlers in the form of physical play, which young children find enjoyable and often requires touch. Whether it's a round of "This Little Piggy" on your toddler's toes, a few minutes of tickling, or some play wrestling with your elementary-aged kid, the brief physical connection and playtime are great. These moments of playful touch will help build your connection with your child while helping them develop a healthy relationship with their bodies and physical affection.

Respecting Boundaries

Now when encouraging the need for more hugs, you must recognize that as your children get older, they may change their minds about how much physical affection they want. While all children are unique, many kids may not like certain types of touch — particularly as they get older or if they have sensory sensitivities. Observe how your child responds and tailor your method as needed. We're not here to make her feel forced into unwanted contact, the aim is to give her good experiences with physical affection.

Positive Changes

If we incorporate more intentional touch into our parenting, I expect that we will see an improvement in our relationship with our children. According to Dr. Darcia Narvaez, a professor of psychology at the University of Notre Dame, "We know affectionate touch shapes children's development as moral agents, their stress reactivity and social competence." When we make time for these small touch points, we are not only expressing love, but helping to build our children's social and emotional development.

Why how touch gives hope in this world of screen

We have come to live in a world where everything is digital, yet physical touch continues to be one of the most crucial things. Touching physically is one of the fastest ways to practice mindfulness and presence that we should engage with our children. Every hug, every encouragement from you with a high-five or gentle touch on the back is not just about helping our child with something difficult; we are connecting to them in that present moment, engaging at so deep of a level — it needs no more explanation than this.

Short, frequent touches form the best basis of safety in our lives and will benefit your children long-term. We are going to go more into mindfulness techniques in the next chapter, but do bear in mind that physical touch can be mindfulness in and of itself as it allows you or your child to come back to the present moment, physically tenderizing yourself or him/her when life gets busy.

Chapter 10

Apart from physical affection, another area of nurture for ourselves and our children is mindfulness. This chapter will show how parents (and kids) can make a few minutes of mindfulness work wonders for family harmony.

The Essence of Mindfulness

Mindfulness is about being in the present moment, aware of your thoughts, feelings, and environment without judgment. In the world today where distractions are a dime a dozen and stress is an unavoidable part of life, it can feel difficult to nudge mindfulness into our routine acts. But the beauty of mindfulness is that it can be practiced in all forms and contexts. In just 5 minutes, we can create a calm, clear and connected feeling that gets carried throughout our day.

Mindfulness for Parents

Mindfulness also has huge benefits for parents. Raising children, maintaining households, sometimes careers can lead to feeling as if we are boiling over and even losing connection. Mindfulness is powerful in any form and at any length, so taking a few moments to practice this will help us get back to center in order that we can feel less stressed and deal with the demands of parenting from a place of calmness. The small stuff Dr. Jon Kabat-Zinn founding director of Mindfulness-Based Stress Reduction: The little moments? They aren't little." So simple yet so true, and another powerful example of a harnessed short moment of mindfulness with children.

Mindful breathing is one of the easiest 5-minute mindfulness exercises for parents to do together. Make a safe space of your own — even if it's just a corner in your room or for a minute you parked before entering the house. Just breathe, close your eyes. Focus on how it feels when air enters and leaves your body. Maybe your mind wanders—when this happens, simply notice and guide your attention back to the breath with no judgment attached. This very easy practice begins to resettle your nervous system, lowers the stress in your body and allows you space to be responsive instead of reactive with what your children need and how they behave.

The body scan is another brief mindfulness tool for parents. Focus on the area starting from the top of your head, slowly moving down through your body and paying attention to areas of tension or pain. When you notice these spaces, picture your breath entering them and letting go of the tension with every out-breath. It allows you to reconnect with your body and is a useful method for noticing and addressing stress before it gets in the way of how you behave towards your kids.

Mindfulness for Kids

Teaching children to be more mindful can measurably affect their emotional control, ability to pay attention, and well-being in general. The key, of course, is to keep these practices fun and age-appropriate. Here is a short 5-minute mindfulness exercise you can do with kids: Mindful Jar Just grab some water in a clear jar with a spoon of glitter. Then shake the jar and observe the movement of glitter. Using TLC to create a glitter jar:13 explain to your child that the glitter represents what thoughts and feelings look like when we are in fight-or-flight mode. Once the glitter has settled down, we have a quieter mind. It creates a visual for them to help them understand and practice letting thoughts and feelings settle on their own.

The activity titled: Superhero Senses game is another fun mindfulness exercise for kids. Encouraging your child to use their super hearing, sight, smell, taste or touch and just pay attention for 1 minute to their environment. It cultivates sensory awareness and the art of being present with a child. For example: You could say, "Use your superpower of hearing; Искусственный интеллект, сделавший самый отдаленный звук ты слышишь, какой? Now, what's the closest?" This is a game that you can play anytime so the potential to transform stressful moments and situations (waiting rooms, long car rides, etc.) into mindfulness practice is massive.

Mindfulness for Families

It allows families to connect with each other deeply if practiced together. One of the easiest ways a family can practice mindfulness together might be to find five minutes throughout your day and sit in a circle, taking it in turns to say one thing you are grateful for, one challenge you are facing, and one hope for the future. This practice helps recognize that we do indeed have an emotional experience as human beings, and at the same time it strengthens family connection using empathy (as the other side of a relation).

You can also make discipline from mindfulness a habit by implementing them in day to day life. You could bring an exercise of mindful eating as part of a meal. Give only one minute of time to focus on the colors, scents, and textures of the food — before eating. It encourages mindfulness, which may result in healthy eating habits and a better appreciation of food.

Consistency is Key

Being mindful takes practice. Like any developing routine, it expects consistency. Try 5 minutes of mindfulness practice a day for you or with your children. You might find a steady practice to be even less natural, so you can increase frequency or duration as they become more second nature.

Mindfulness in Parenting

Perhaps the greatest advantage of mindfulness for parents is that it allows us to respond rather than react in hard situations. Daniel Siegel,a clinical professor of psychiatry at the UCLA School of Medicine, calls it the "pause." "If we slow down, we are not reacting to the initial impulse which is typically a negative one," he says. When we infuse a few minutes of mindfulness into our day, we are developing this capacity to pause — to respond rather than react. This translates into more mindful and compassionate parenting choices.

Mindfulness has additional benefits for children in addition to emotional regulation. Recordings have suggested that regular mindfulness practice can increase concentration and attention, promote social abilities, and even enhance educational achievements. The Journal of Child and Family Studies published a study that proved children would significantly benefit from executive functioning after participating in a mindfulness program by showing improved impulse control and cognitive flexibility.

Conclusion

So, as we can wrap this section on mindfulness for both parents and kids — really even the smallest amounts of mindfulness can change family life. These 5-minute practices, woven into our everyday lives, create opportunities for calm and connection that can change everything in our parenting experience. Bear in mind that you are aiming for progress, not perfection. Whenever family members engage in a mindful moment, it is a stride towards a more balanced, conscious and harmonious existence.

Next up, some ideas on how these relatively short practices and purposeful moments can carry into other aspects of parenting (because fostering responsibility among our kiddos? Mindfulness simply coalesces itself to a foundation of presence and awareness that you will use in raising kids to understand accountability and independence which we will address next chapter.

Chapter 11

Now switching gears from the mindfulness practices I talked about in Part 1, but speaking to another important aspect of parenting: a sense of responsibility. One important trait you want them to develop as they mature into competent, self-sufficient adults is responsibility. The good news? It doesn't have to be difficult, or take forever. With our 5-minute parenting in mind, we will talk about how short and consistent moments can go a long way in building responsibility and autonomy. Consider for a moment spending only a couple of minutes each day giving your child little chores to do or letting him/her participate in decisions. Just by doing this can add a sense of ownership to their responsibility. Incorporating these brief yet powerful moments into your day can allow you to support and instill valuable life skills in your child without the need for an extensive time commitment.

Breaking Down Responsibility

Responsibility is scary for parents and kids. Stressed out parents are concerned about the holiday season being overwhelming, and finding that fine line of putting kids to work or giving them time to themselves. It is possible that children would be under pressure due to expectations or challenged to assume new responsibilities. The secret is to split the process into 5 minute modules that we can easily slot into our every day routine. This gives a platform for stable, step by step development of accountability without acting as a focal point of pressure or pushback.

A 5-Minute Chore Of Your Choice

First, consider implementing a system of 5-minute chores. It starts to bring children into family organization by having things that are fun and simple. A 5-minute chore system is so beautiful because it is short and sweet. This time-limiting approach eliminates the fear we tend to associate with chores, while still reinforcing one feels good having done something productive.

Write down a list of tasks that each child can do that will only take five minutes and is appropriate for their age. This could vary from cleaning up toys to feeding a pet to setting the table with younger children. Middle school-aged kids can be given tasks of greater responsibility, like a speed cleanup of a certain room (5 minutes max to erase the evidence), wipe counters in the bathrooms, or sort laundry. Keep the $5 worth of tasks in under 5 minutes to avoid creating frustration while keeping motivation high!

After determining your, set up a simple chart or digital app to monitor and do rotations of roles. It also adds fairness and introduces kids to many household chores gradually. You might try using a timer to make the 5 minutes more tangible, and inject some fun challenges. The notion of beating the clock turns chores into a game, rather than seeing chores as a dreaded obligation which many kids resentfully take.

The aim, according to psychologist Dr. Laura Markham, is "to help kids feel like an important part of the family." The key is to accept chores as part of family life and adopt a positive attitude about them: when children notice an attachment from parents about something, they tend to follow suit without putting up a struggle." Short, easy tasks provide our children a sense of success, give them positive associations with being responsible.

Took some accountability blink out lessons

Now, beyond chores, let us look into how we can serve up short lessons in accountability within the flow of day-to-day interactions. These lessons aren't formal sit-down at the table kind of things, they can be weaved into conversation and activity. Ex: Instead of saying, "Put your toys away" or putting it away yourself, explain what will happen if they do not pick up after themselves. Maybe you say "I see the toys you used are still all over the floor. What do you think that does to our family, huh? Showing them walking in their own lane ... "What can happen if someone falls over?

This short exchange shames them into thinking critically about the effect their actions (or inaction) have on others. A minor yet effective method to instill accountability in a relationship. Likewise, when your child actually does a task or follows through on a commitment, give them specific acknowledgement. Something as straightforward as, "Hey, I saw that you hang your backpack up without me telling you to." Which reinforces positive behaviors and connects them to responsibility: "That really helps our front entryway stay tidy, and it also shows such great responsibility.

Natural Consequences

The use of natural consequences is another good method of teaching accountability. Let children feel the consequences of their choices when safe and reasonable. If a kid leaves their lunch behind, don't race to the school with it. Treat it as a 5-minute learning session instead. Talk about how they felt not to have lunch, come up with ideas to not let this happen again, and maybe collaborate on a morning checklist for next time.

Natural consequences are what Dr. Jane Nelsen calls it in her book Positive Discipline, where your children learn from doing, rather than lecturing them on the subject. Parental rescuing robs children of learning experiences through the natural consequences of their actions." When we allow for these moments and make sure to briefly but meaningfully discuss them, we reinforce a greater sense of accountability for our own children.

Independence Provided in Short Bursts

Another great way to promote responsibility is through quick, independent tasks. The aim is to help them become more independent while still giving guidance when required. Begin with items that your child can do alone, or at least without your help — even if they only presently do so with your assistance. This can be as simple as getting their school bag ready, picking out their clothes for the following day or preparing a light meal.

Introduce these tasks slowly, one at a time, and spend only a few minutes each day facilitating your child as he/she begins to learn how to take responsibility for completing the task. So, take 5 minutes just demonstrating to your child how you make a bed step by step. Give less and less help each day for the next few days, always reassuring them that they are making progress.

Children learn real-life skills from completing these tasks as well as a sense of confidence in being able to perform them. That confidence often translates into other areas of their life and motivates them to embrace new challenges and responsibilities. As Dr. Marilyn Price-Mitchell, developmental psychologist and researcher, says: "When children gain independence, they take charge of their own actions. Through this, they cultivate an awareness of their internal whys & will learn to make decisions that are in alignment with their well-being and the well being of others.

Conclusion

Developing a sense of responsibility is not something that happens overnight, it takes time and practice. So along the path there are going to be obstacles and frustrations — those things are just part of learning. 5 Minutes: It keeps us focused on responsibility but does not let it get too crazy for either parent or child.

They say, even small and steady actions can make noteworthy changes. We set the stage in bulk by establishing a 5-minute chore system, delivering fast lessons on accountability, and encouraging independence through short tasks.

Chapter 12

Since we are transitioning into moving our children out of independence, let us not baby them and instead guide their creativity. Creativity helps improve problem-solving, self-expression and cognitive development skills in general. In this chapter, we will instantaneously uncover big 5-minutes-a-day tips that are perfect for the busiest parents to jumpstart your child's imagination development.

This is the beauty of creation, anyone can implement it. It doesn't cost a lot of money and you don't need to set up anything fancy. But creativity flourishes with richness and impulse; it is highly aligned with our 5-minute parenting homeschool. So, whether it be through spontaneous art projects, playing make-believe games or simply indulging in creative thinking during daily life experiences, this also nurtures a passion to engage in more formal creative outlet activities later on.

5-Minute Art Projects

These minuscule creative activities offer a little thematic, artistic exploration for your child that you can slip into their daily life.

Scribble story: Give your child a piece of paper and a crayon, set the timer for 30 seconds and ask them to scribble without lifting the crayon. Encourage them to search for shapes or objects in the scribble, then color those images with markers or colored pencils. This activity is seriously so creative and encourages visual perception and dexterity.

Nature Collage: Wait two minutes and look for small items in nature such as leaves, twigs or pebbles on a brief spur outside or in your garden. After that, set down three minutes for your child to stick these items onto a sheet of paper or cardboard to make a nature collage. This generates both creativeness and excitement for the natural creations of the world as well as awareness of how these figures occupy space.

One-Minute Sculpture — Give your child a small piece of playdough or clay and set a timer and get him to sculpt something in just one minute. This is an exciting pressure, as there's a time limit and you have to think on your feet! Use the remaining four minutes to talk about their creation, how they came up with this idea and compliment them on their initiative. This hikes fine motor, spatial reasoning and verbal expression skills.

Quick Imagination Exercises

Such activities stimulate your kid's brain &_drive them to think creatively in short intervals.

What If? : Ask your child a goofy question, like if trees had legs, would they be able to walk? "What if cats could talk?" Allow them a minute to reflect, and then have four minutes to offer their creative answers. This is a creative thinking exercise that develops verbal skills, and encourages logical analytical mind.

Story in a Bag: Place three to five random objects you can find around the house into a bag. Have your child look at the items for a minute, then spend four minutes writing a short story to include all of the objects. This promotes narrative and object association, out-of-the-box thinking!

Multiple Uses: Pick any common everyday object — a paper clip, a shoe, anything — and ask your child to think of all the possible alternative uses for it in three minutes. Use the last two minutes to talk about their ideas, and maybe contribute a few of your own. This activity encourages divergent thinking, which is an important aspect of creativity.

Cultivating Creative Moments Throughout the Day

You don't have to schedule things for your child, to integrate creativity in their life. Some suggestions on how to include it as part of your daily regimen:

Create a new meal: Ask your child to create a recipe consisting of three ingredients from the fridge? It can be unrealistic to cook their creation, but thinking through flavors and plating provides a creative exploration.

In the Car and Waiting: Switch up I Spy Scavenge for Challenges:Get your child to explain things in unique manners go! Instead of I spy something red, try I spy something that looks like a sleeping dragon. It promotes relatively the same kind of imagination as well as figurative language skills.

Undersea Adventure → bath time story: get some bath toys, take your time making up a little adventure under the sea with whoever you bring in to play. This makes bath time fun and encourages story-telling skills and imaginative play.

Collaborative Bedtime Stories — Launch a collaborative bedtime story in which you start with one sentence, and your child adds the next. For five minutes switch back and forth telling a different story every night. Not only does this ignite creativity but it also reinforces your relationship and encourages a positive experience around bedtime.

Supporting Creativity

These 5 min creativity sparks are not intended for masterpieces, but the process of creating and being creative, and enhancing/improving creativity is what makes them meaningful. In the words of Pablo Picasso, "Every child is an artist. The question is how to keep being an artist as adults. When we regularly offer short, but high quality creative experiences, we allow our children's natural artistic souls to flourish and be able to sustain that creativity into their adult years.

It is important to have an atmosphere that enables and promotes creativeness. Encourage your child for their creative work, hang them up somewhere at home and be genuinely interested in their imaginations. Children who believe their creativity is appreciated will want to embrace and explore that creativity further.

Be a Model Yourself for Creativity. Show your child that you are an active creator, doodling in the sketchbook or mixing a new approximation of your favorite recipe, and maybe even solving a new household problem. Children are always watching, and if they see you incorporating creativity in your everyday life, they will follow suit.

Conclusion

This is the final section of our spark of creativity segment, and in hitting this point, it becomes evident that such fast creative exercises not only provide an artistic output. They develop skills in effective problem solving, greater confidence, improved communication and great bonding opportunities. Focusing on creativity for just 5 minutes a day is an investment in your child's brain development, emotional health and social skills.

Next, we will discuss ways to build healthy habits through bite sized opportunities with our kids. As time goes on we will learn that just as creativity can be instilled in small moments, so can our physical wellness and awareness of nutrition. 5-Minute Parenting — Small Actions, Big Impact in Our KidsThe 5 Minute Parenting Journey Continues | by Leo & Pearls

Chapter 13

Having discussed the role of creativity in our day-to-day events, we now shift to another vital area in family life: Health & Wellness. With life getting so busy these days, finding time to stay healthy is really a challenge. But with the 5-Minute Parenting Philosophy, we can weave critical wellness practices into our daily activities without overburdening our calendars.

Quick Physical Activities

Regular exercise is an essential component of any healthy person—and incorporating activity into family life does not have to be time-consuming or complicated. A few minutes of brisk, energetic movement with a kid can provide real dividends for adults and children alike.

Morning Family Stretch: A quick family stretch session to start your day. And as you and your kids reach up high to the sky, bend down low to touch your toes, and twist from side-to-side, not only are you waking your bodies up but in reality you are also kicking off a great start to the day! It can help increase flexibility, ramp up circulation and sharpen mental acuity — all before breakfast is on the table.

Dance Party: If you want something more intense, do a five-minute dance party. Choose a song that you like with an upbeat rhythm, and get everyone dancing. Not to mention, dancing is great cardio and lifts your spirits. As the great dancer Martha Graham said, "dance is the secret language of the soul". Encouraging your family to get up and dance — even just for a couple of minutes — encourages everyone to be happy and connected whilst staying active.

The Animal Walk Game is a short and effective physical activity animal walk game. Get your kids to move around like a different animal for 30 seconds at a time. They could bounce like a kangaroo, creep like a snake or trot like a horse. Besides being a killer workout for several muscle groups, balancing also promotes coordination and often ends with fits of laughter – something good for the emotional well-being, too! They are not trying to develop Olympians; they want their kids to enjoy moving and understand that it is a need in life.

How to Prepare Quick and Healthy Snack

Nutrition: As we say, "you are what you eat," and when it comes to growing children, this is even more true. We simply sometimes do not have the time to cook up healthy meals, at least that's how it feels. This is where you want to prepare quick healthy snacks. You can whip up wholesome, energizing snacks for your family in five minutes or less.

Rainbow Plate Challenge: Take five minutes to support your little ones in choosing and arranging fruits and vegetables of different colors on a single plate. This makes healthy eating enjoyable and guarantees a range of micronutrients. Red for strawberries to vitamin C, orange for carrots to beta-carotene, green cucumber to hydrate—every color has its health benefits. While you are preparing this snack together, take a minute to talk about how our bodies benefit from a variety of colors in our food.

Yogurt Parfait Bar: Provide plain yogurt and some diced fruit along with granola or nuts. Family members can build their own parfaits in five minutes. In one cup, this snack is a protein, probiotics, vitamins and fiber powerhouse. When parents let their children choose their own food, they become independent and tend to have a liking for healthy foods.

Veggie Dippers Station: For those who prefer more of a savory snack option, the "veggie dippers" station features◇◇◇ Adapt this as per your liking what vegetables do you like to eat so cut down a few like bell peppers and other have some celery or maybe cherry tomatoes. Pair these with hummus or a simple home-prepared dip of Greek yogurt and herbs. It's a great way to provide nutrients and teach kids with exposure towards veggies from an early age.

As your child makes the snacks, take those few minutes to have a short conversation about body awareness and health. Example questions: How do you think this food benefits our bodies? Meaning of some health or "What does it mean to be in good health" These quick chats set up a lifetime of health awareness.

Promoting mental and emotional well-being

Your Health Is Not Just Physical Of course, mental and emotional health matter just as much, especially in the high-stress environment we live in today. Spend five minutes every day doing a family "gratitude circle". Everyone goes around and shares something they are grateful for about their body or health. This is a very simple and positive activity that plays a great role in promoting positive vibes, appreciating your body as it is, and paying attention to your health.

Body Scan Meditation — Body scan meditation in five minutes is another fast approach to overall wellness. Have your children lie down in a cozy position and then gradually guide their focus to parts of their body — from toes all the way to the top of their head. This is tons of body awareness, stress relief and sleep —three essentials for good health.

Laughter: A Powerful Promoter of Wellness — Never underestimate the power of laughter in your life. Take five minutes to swap some jokes or funny stories. It can strengthen the immune system, relieve pain and reduce stress. If laughter is the best medicine, then it is also a medicine you can and should incorporate into your wellness routine every day.

Conclusion

And as we wrap up this section on health and wellness habits, please remember that these simple five minute practices, when done consistently will change the whole well being of your family. You are doing the groundwork for life long healthy habits by incorporating some quick physical activities, preparing healthier food options and encouraging discussions surrounding health.

Join us next time, when we impact the world of technology and its place in parenting today. This is about how to balance screen time and use some digital tools to strengthen the knots of family ties, ending with our 5 minutes approach. Now, the jump from health habits to tech-smart parenting may seem jarring but in our digital age, technology use is quickly becoming a core element of the definition of healthy family lifestyle.

Chapter 14

Technology has now taken a central role in our children's lives, especially in this digital world. The students gain significant advantage through technology that involves the utmost struggle for every parent living in the present age — providing optimal human experience complemented with engagement outside of electronic media. Parenting in the Digital Age: A Five-Minute GuideFor Parenting Basics Including How to Control Screen Time, Teaching Digital Literacy, and Getting Tech Right for Meaningful Engagement after Explaining What Each Form of Technology is For byFREE Book PreviewThe 5 Second RuleGet an exclusive sneak peek of this book right now.

Managing Screen Time

Dividing screen time into 5-minute increments doesn't feel like it should work well. But again, we're not talking about screen use of only 5 minutes here – rather how do we develop healthier digital behavior using short, targeted techniques?

5-Minute warning: Before you are ready to switch off a screen, tell your child five minutes before. This is just enough time to finish processing whatever they are doing, and prepare themselves mentally for the change. Inquire as to, "What is the most amazing thing you have seen? In these last few minutes, "What do you want to achieve?" This signals engagement on your part with their digital world and promotes the opportunity to reflect upon the time spent on their devices.

5 Minute Break from Screen: Do a break for 5 minutes whenever you use the screen for every 30 minutes. Take the time to stretch, gaze at something far away (excellent for eye health), or perform a quick workout. This practice further helps me to keep the perception that technology usage must always be countered with real-world engagements.

Tech Check Before Tech Hand Out (5 Minutes) — After getting a device or power on the TV, talk for five minutes about what they are going to do, watch or play. This one-minute conversation redirects screenew time from aimlessness and online drifting toward something more intentional and focused.

Digital Literacy

Digital literacy is very important — but it does not take hour-long lectures. Brief lessons over watering will go a long way to help children learn how to navigate opioid day.

Online Advertising: In the event that your child comes across an advertisement while in an app, use 5 minutes to explain how online advertising works. Briefly we talked about how the internet works in terms of targeted ads, data collection, and why you need to filter content and think critically when you consume anything online.

Online Safety: If your child is contacted by someone not on their friend list in any of the apps, tell them you want to talk for a moment about online privacy and dangers associated with talking to people we don't know. Lessons like these are easier to stick to in a timely manner.

Fact-checking: If your child comes excited with some cool new "fact" they read online, use the next 5 minutes to teach them how to check information from credible sources. It instills critical thinking and questioning online information — one of the most important skills in times of misinformation!

Technology that Matters

Technology can create genuine engagement when used with thoughtfulness.

Short weekly video chats: Chat with far-flung family members over video for 5 minutes. Start a mini storytime, display something they've done recently, or just stop by to say hi. These are short visits that maintain the family connection.

5-Min Family Quests: Access a brain teaser, riddle or trivia question online and solve it together as a family. This encourages families to bond and solve problems together.

Educational App Sessions — Children will Be Using iPads in the Classroom: Mini lesson of five mins regarding a new concept in math, science, or language (there is an abundance of apps here; pick one that has won awards for quality) This makes passive screen time interactive learning through your engagement.

Digital Art Sessions – You and your child can use a drawing app for 5-minute digital art sessions where you draw a quick sketch or do some pure "artwork" together. This fosters creativity and teaches fundamental skills in the digital world.

Modeling Healthy Tech Habits

Our kids tend to learn more from our actions than words. Practice what you preach in terms of healthy tech habits. Give a 5-minute tech check-in of your own to show mindful use of technology. Before reaching for your phone or laptop, ask yourself whether that action is really needed. Use a narration with your child about it "Just going to check my email really fast in case I got an important message from your teacher."

Conclusion

Tech-savvy parenting does not condemn technology or impose blanket rules. Whatever that means for each individual family — whether it's complete digital detox or mindful engagement with technology and the internet — focusing on what works best for your family as opposed to what might be ideal for others. We can be intentional with technology with these 5 minute strategies to help our children at this stage of their life.

In summary, as we reach the end of this chapter, it is clear that even tiny but repeated efforts can go a long way in shaping how our kids will engage with technology in the future and make sure their relationship with it is on healthy footing. These short 5-minute actions—monitoring screen time, educating on digital literacy, and purposeful participation—can impact healthy online behavior. Next, we will see how these quick but profound moments can be more than just online adventures and evolve into lifelong family traditions.

Chapter 15

While completing our course in the world of 5-minute parenting, we uncover the indelible mark made by family traditions. Even such short practices serve the purpose of connecting families across generations. In this chapter, we will explore how the most basic of rituals can create a strong experience of belonging, stability, and family identity together — your family unit. Whether it is a short game night once every week, a bedtime story that has been told for generations, these micro-moments linger and help create everlasting memories and tighten your family's unique structure. These traditions will not only enhance your family life, but they will create connections that echo for generations!

Creating 5-Minute Rituals

The art of simplicity with significant moments is to create daily or weekly rituals limited to between 5 mins. They don't have to be long—in fact, the shorter and more meaningful they are the better, as even these practices can help form an anchor around which your family life can continue to turn at a predictable pace that children naturally crave. Just think about a family huddle that takes place daily — everyone meets together for just five minutes, sharing what they are going to do that day, or what went well. Those few seconds can be the start of a good day and get those precious family relationships into full swing.

One family I worked with did a "rose and thorn" at the dinner table each night. In these moments, the family members share their rose (the best part of their day) and then each thorn (the worst part of their day.) Not only does this simple practice promote open dialogue, but it helps kids learn how to process their experiences and feelings. As one mother noted, "In those few minutes we all learn so much about each other's lives. We used to have it a few times a week, but now we have it every day. These little rituals can turn ordinary moments into chances for bonding, hence enriching and enlivening family life!

And your weekly rituals can wield equal power. In time, a Sunday evening game night or a Saturday morning pancake breakfast or even a Friday afternoon dance party can become a family tradition that everyone anticipates. They don't have to be fancy events; the important thing is that it's consistent and enjoyed together. One father I counseled started the "Wacky Walk Wednesdays" by taking 5 minutes to walk around the block with his children after dinner — but had to do it in the silliest way possible. He said, "It's just five minutes but jaida chare dunavor aai see afu putra."

The best part about these 5-minute traditions is that they are completely doable for even the busiest families. All you need to commit to is setting aside a small bit of time from your calendar on a regular basis; they don't take much in the way of planning or resources. {Note: If you want some guidance on how to balance "spiking" creative projects with routine structured ones, check out my free eBook here.} As family therapist William Doherty so aptly puts it, "Rituals are to relationships what containers are to liquids. They keep us from falling apart when the living gets messy.

Celebrating Milestones

An important principle of building family traditions is to mark milestones either in a speedy manner or with a pinch of creativity. As you so well know, these days it's way too easy to overlook milestones. However, spending just five minutes to acknowledge these moments can make a world of difference in a child's life. Image: Random living room dance party for a good grade, special high-five combo for losing a tooth, or family round of cheers bumps for mineral water. These little celebrations not only inject some joy in your day-to-day routine, but they also help create an atmosphere of recognition and support within your family. When you get into the habit of celebrating the smallest victories, you program your children to keep those memories close to their hearts along with a sense of pride and belonging for many years!

A great mom I worked with started a "victory lap" tradition. Whenever one of the family accomplished something — any accomplishment, large or small — they would take a victory lap around the dining room table while everybody else cheered and applauded. There will be time taken — a minute or two, she said, but worth it when everyone feels great and proud.

These lapses in original celebrations serve several purposes. They bolster positive behaviors and accomplishments, provide confidence-boosting compliments, and form a healthy relationship to success and hard work. They also teach children how to honor others' successes in a loving, family-friendly manner.

In the first week of working together, we want to establish a couple of customs that are important for our team, yet easy and not time-consuming to do.

Creating short but meaningful family rituals may be the best thing you can leave behind as a parent. And these traditions are the tales your kids tell their own children, the moments that will bring a smile to their face many years from now. It is simply about discovering traditions that align with your family values and personality.

For example, an environmentally-minded family could have a 5-minutes "Earth Hero of the Week" where they share a single action they took that week to help save our planet. A family that emphasizes education might create a "Word of the Day" tradition, taking five minutes during breakfast to learn and use a new word. A family with musical interests could have a "Song Share," where each person can play one song and the others get to hear that week's favorite.

I learned of a particularly touching tradition from a family where the father was frequently moving them for work. They invented a ritual called Heart Home. Every time they would move to a new place, they spent 5 minutes in the empty new house together standing in a circle with their arms around each other. And they would close their eyes and the mother would say, "The place we are together is our heart home." It was a simple yet powerful tradition that brought the children value because no matter where they were in the world, they had something to hold on to.

Note that the most significant rituals are usually pretty simple and inexpensive. Like a goodnight kiss with a special phrase, or secret handshake, or saying "I love you" in a certain way that turns into family traditions. The days are long but the years are short as author — paper collaborating Gretchen Rubin says. These 5-minute customs remind us to maximize on those ephemeral years when children are home, weaving a textile of family & shared experiences and memories.

Adapting Traditions

Keep in mind that consistency is key to tradition but also flexible. Especially as your family changes when children get older, you may need to change some traditions or try a new one all together. That 5-minute bedtime story may become a 5-minute conversation about the day when your kids hit their teenage years. Although the specific activities will change, the spirit of connecting and shared experiences needs to remain.

Conclusion

These 5-minute practices are a great way to turn things into family traditions that ultimately lead to stronger family bonds, memories, and lessons in the values you find important. These minor but meaningful traditions provide children with a feeling of self and community that they will take with them into adulthood. So as you venture further into this journey of parenthood, remember that it is not the size and texture of your traditions that matters, but instead the love, consistency, and breadth of meaning that underlies them. It takes just five minutes a day, yet you can leave a legacy of connection and belonging for generations to come. So, relish in these minutes—every single one is a new thread to the vast tapestry of familial love and time spent together!

Book Summary

In The 5-Minute Parent: Small Habits, Big Impact, we've explored how small moments with our kids can have a really big impact. Between subjective lessons from morning rituals to bedtime bonding; to emotional check-ins and micro-learning moments, we learned that it is quality over quantity. Such relatively minor interactions can help us develop better relationships, nurture emotional intelligence and build more positive effects in our kids' lives.

These are not strategies that require hours of time each day; you will see from the pages in this book that great parenting doesn't need to take much time at all. Rather, it is about maximizing what we have in each instant and making even the mundane a time to connect with others, learn something new or grow. Integration of these 5-minute habits into our daily routines will facilitate providing the perfect ecosystem in which children grow up having developed emotionally, cognitively and physically.

That's one of the most powerful takeaways from this method: It's easy. We can all devote or at least manufacture five minutes here or there to engage with our kids. Little investments of time and attention compound over days, weeks, and years to create an infrastructure for a child that will guide them toward a sense of safety in the world, the belief that they have value as a person, an understanding of their place (or lack thereof) in relation to others. And of course, they make life easier for us parents too, so we can be present with our children and navigate stress while finding pleasure in the little things with the family.

On this note, ending the journey with a recap of the importance is not about perfection but taking steps towards progress in becoming a 5-minute parent. It is about finding the movement of your heart to be more present, intentional, and connected in the time we have with our kids. If we continue to adopt these small ways of living, it can make a significant difference in establishing healthy, loving relationships helping our children stand through this world throughout their lives.

In the end, it is these eternal passing moments — A laugh shared-A hug given-A conversation had; That our kids will remember and take with them from childhood to adulthood. So let us savor these fleeting moments because they have the potential to fill our children's hearts and memories for a lifetime.

www.ingramcontent.com/pod-product-compliance
Lightning Source LLC
Chambersburg PA
CBHW061735250726
48657CB00002B/931